# HIGH-INTEREST STEAM

# COSMETICS

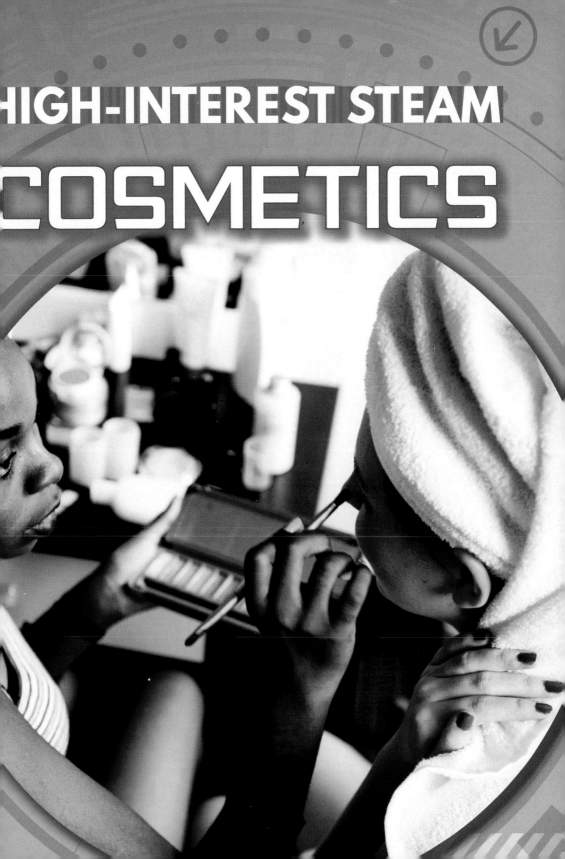

# HIGH-INTEREST STEAM

AUTOMOBILES

COSMETICS

DRONES

ENVIRONMENT

FASHION

GAMING

MUSIC

SMARTPHONES

SOCIAL MEDIA

SPORTS

# HIGH-INTEREST STEAM

# COSMETICS

**MARY DEAN**

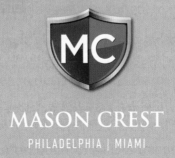

## MASON CREST
PHILADELPHIA | MIAMI

**MASON CREST**
PO Box 221876
Hollywood, FL 33022
(866) MCP-BOOK (toll-free) • www.masoncrest.com

Copyright © 2022 by Mason Crest, an imprint of National Highlights, Inc. All rights reserved.

First printing
9 8 7 6 5 4 3 2 1
ISBN (hardback) 978-1-4222-4518-7
ISBN (series) 978-1-4222-4516-3
ISBN (ebook) 978-1-4222-7287-9

Library of Congress Cataloging-in-Publication Data

Names: Dean, Mary, author.
Title: Cosmetics / Mary Dean.
Description: Hollywood, FL : Mason Crest, [2022] | Series: High-interest steam |
    Includes bibliographical references and index.
Identifiers: LCCN 2020003295 | ISBN 9781422245187 (hardback) |
    ISBN 9781422272879 (ebook)
Subjects: LCSH: Beauty, Personal–Juvenile literature. |
    Cosmetics–Juvenile literature. | Cosmetics–Physiological
    effects–Juvenile literature.
Classification: LCC RA778 .D278 2022 | DDC 646.7/2–dc23
LC record available at https://lccn.loc.gov/2020003295

Developed and Produced by National Highlights, Inc.
Editor: Andrew Luke
Production: Crafted Content, LLC

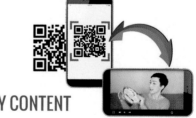

## QR CODES AND LINKS TO THIRD-PARTY CONTENT

# CONTENTS

# KEY ICONS TO LOOK FOR

**Words to Understand:** These words with their easy-to-understand definitions will increase the readers' understanding of the text while building vocabulary skills.

**Sidebars:** This boxed material within the main text allows readers to build knowledge, gain insights, explore possibilities, and broaden their perspectives by weaving together additional information to provide realistic and holistic perspectives.

**Educational Videos:** Readers can view videos by scanning our QR codes, providing them with additional educational content to supplement the text. Examples include news coverage, moments in history, speeches, iconic sports moments, and much more!

**Text-Dependent Questions:** These questions send the reader back to the text for more careful attention to the evidence presented there.

**Research Projects:** Readers are pointed toward areas of further inquiry connected to each chapter. Suggestions are provided for projects that encourage deeper research and analysis.

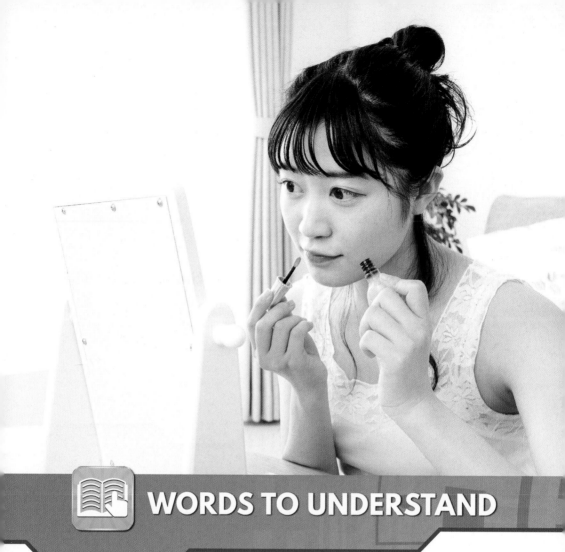

## WORDS TO UNDERSTAND

**chemistry**—the science that deals with the composition and properties of substances and various elementary forms of matter

**cosmetics**—superficial measures to make something appear better, more attractive, or more impressive

**emollients**—ingredients that soothe or soften skin and seal in moisture by slowing water evaporation

**emulsions**—mixtures of two or more liquids in which one is present as droplets distributed throughout the other

**Kohl**—an ancient cosmetic made by grinding stibnite

**psychology**—the science of the mind or of mental states and processes

# CHAPTER 1

# SCIENCE
## IN COSMETICS

At first glance, it might seem like science and **cosmetics** have very little in common. After all, it doesn't take a rocket scientist to contour foundation or be a pro at wing eyeliner. However, a deeper look reveals that there are tons of scientific actions going on behind the scenes during the creation and application of makeup, skincare products, and the like. There is even a branch called cosmetic science that studies the effects that beauty-focused products have on the body. Who knew that the process of getting made up could be just as much science as it is art?

## A SHORT HISTORY OF COSMETICS

Long before there was MAC, Clinique, and Neutrogena, our distant ancestors were crafting cosmetics in an attempt to improve their skin and appearance. Although many people think of cosmetics and makeup as synonymous, many kinds of cosmetics don't involve

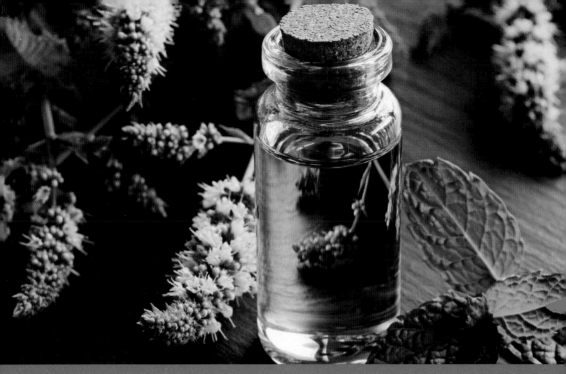

*The ancient Egyptians used peppermint oil, among other things, to help mask their body odor.*

something like coloring the face. These include lotions, bath oils, hair dyes, contact lenses, and nail polish.

The first recorded use of cosmetics dates back thousands of years to ancient Egypt. Not only did they use lily, peppermint, and cedar oils to camouflage the smell of sweat brought on by the desert heat, they also created creams to protect their skin from the dry winds. This isn't surprising since the Egyptians were trendsetters in lots of areas like writing, agriculture, and architecture.

Centuries after Cleopatra used ground-up beetles to paint her lips, tribes in southern Europe began to tattoo their skin. Mesopotamian women in what is now known as Iraq started to make their own perfume and skincare lines. Across the Himalayan Mountains, the Chinese made painting one's fingernails popular, and the Japanese were lightening their skin with natural powders. Grecian women wore fake eyebrows made of ox hair (what a fashion

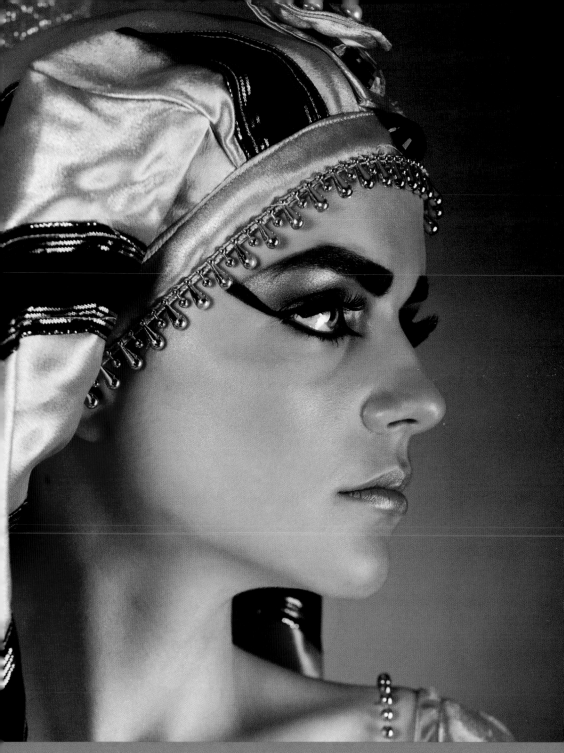

*This model is dressed like an ancient Egyptian, wearing heavy eye makeup as depicted in ancient drawings.*

statement) and crafted lipstick out of clay. Roman men were dying their hair blond while the women of the era were healing pimples with butter and flour. They even used sheep blood to change the color of their nails!

All of this happened in the time BCE, but even after the Common Era began, cosmetics continued to play a huge role in society.

Solid lipstick was invented during the 900s. Queen Elizabeth of Hungary ordered the creation of the first modern perfume in the 1300s. Like many other cosmetics made in the distant past, the uses were as much medicinal as they were for beauty purposes. Queen Elizabeth's "Hungary water" was made from alcohol and natural elements such as thyme, rosemary, lavender, lemon, mint, and sage. It helped relieve headaches and ringing in the ears and was considered a "cure-all" since it treated various illnesses.

The Egyptians also used cosmetics in a scientific way—to help ward off sickness. Famous for wearing chic clothing and intricate jewelry, it is easy to assume that their thick, black eye makeup was just another fashion statement. However, scientists have recently discovered that the **Kohl** used to create this bold eyeliner actually protected their eyes from infections and the glare of the hot desert sun. Females weren't the only ones who used paint for their lips. In the Roman age, men of high social status often put lipstick on to prove their rank.

Unfortunately, not all cosmetics were created through safe and scientifically sound methods. Another famous royal, England's Queen Elizabeth, I popularized the act of painting one's face, neck, and hands with a mixture called Venetian ceruse. The Queen believed that the use of this early cosmetic concoction made her more beautiful. Because this "mask of youth" was lead-based, the paste caused severe skin damage, hair loss, and even death for many of the 18th-century women who applied it. The Queen herself died at the age of sixty-nine wearing a full inch of makeup. Although there are many rumored reasons for her passing, scientists and historians now believe it was due to blood poisoning caused by the ceruse.

It wasn't until the early 1900s that people began to worry about the chemical composition of these cosmetic concoctions they were applying to their bodies and regulatory practices were put into place. Of course, this didn't stop every unhealthy practice from continuing.

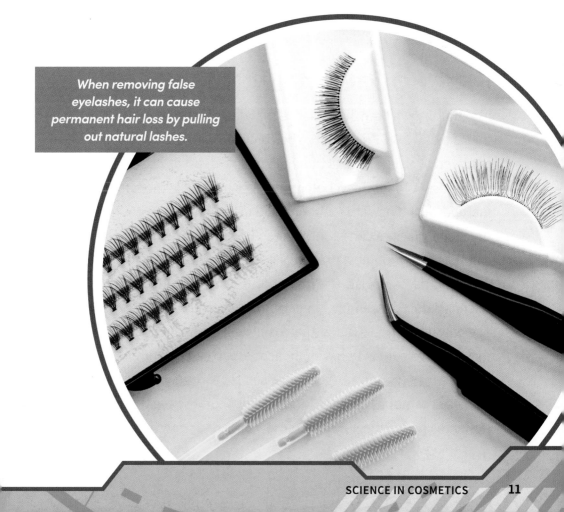

When removing false eyelashes, it can cause permanent hair loss by pulling out natural lashes.

Around 1915, to remove wrinkles on their faces instantly, people were using skin creams made from the radioactive element radium. In the 1920s and 1930s, the "tan" look emerged and caused people to look for products to make themselves darker instead of lighter, even at the expense of their health. Even today, women use chemical peels that can cause serious burns, tattoo their eyebrows, and add false eyelashes that can cause permanent hair loss by pulling out natural lashes when they are removed.

This raises an important question: Why have women (and men) been using products to enhance their looks since the beginning of time, especially when this usage can be expensive and dangerous? It turns out that the answer to this question has its roots in science as well.

## PSYCHOLOGY AND COSMETICS

**Psychology** is a branch of science that deals with why we do the things that we do. This is not to be confused with the treatment rendered by psychologists that help people deal with personal problems. Academic psychology involves training in the scientific method, including data gathering and measurement. Even though psychology lacks a commonly agreed upon body of knowledge, it can still be considered a branch of science for a few reasons. First, academic psychologists use many of the same methods as traditional scientists do. For example, they hypothesize and conduct experiments. The only difference is rather than using test tubes and microscopes, they observe human behavior in response to certain stimuli.

You may (or may not) be surprised to learn that most people who use cosmetics do so to influence how others see them. The desire to change the way others view us is one that we aren't even aware of, so don't judge makeup wearers too harshly. Scientifically speaking, it seems to work. Studies have shown that cosmetic use can change the perceptions of others about the user.

If you look at the use of beauty products over time and in all cultures, you'll find that cosmetics are universally used to do a few different things. The first is to make a face symmetrical since symmetry is subconsciously connected to beauty (we will learn more about this during the math section). The other reasons for cosmetic use are eclectic but generally involve making skin tone even, eyes darker, cheeks pinker, and lips redder.

According to the Association for Psychological Science, having darker skin around the lips and the eyes is a sign of femininity and fertility and naturally seen as attractive. Because makeup hides

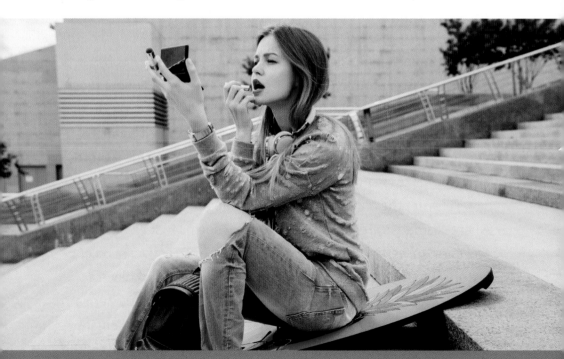

*Red is universally regarded as the most attractive lipstick color due to the contrast it creates.*

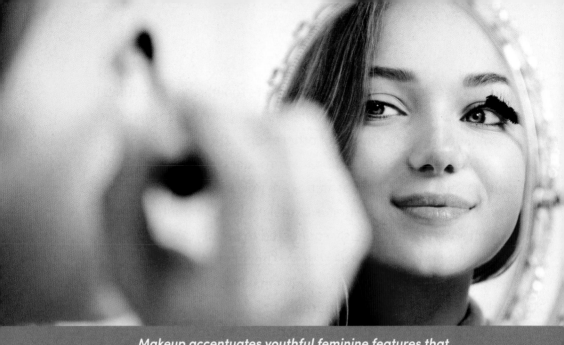

*Makeup accentuates youthful feminine features that men tend to find attractive.*

wrinkles while darkening these areas, it creates a contrast that makes those who use it look younger. Biologically speaking, youth tends to equal beauty. But why is this?

The answer dates back to the most primitive days of humans when to be young and healthy meant you'd be able to carry on the family line. Being evolutionarily attracted to youth helps carry on the human species. Makeup plays up these youthful feminine features and thus makes women more attractive to men.

This isn't the only example of psychological perception change where cosmetics are involved. Although it seems that wearing makeup causes women to be viewed as more attractive, in recent history studies have shown that it can bring about workplace trouble. This is especially true when women who wear cosmetics have female bosses as cosmetic use tends to cause these female bosses to feel more suspicious, threatened, and even jealous of the cosmetic users.

Here are a few more discoveries that scientists and psychology experts have made while studying beauty and cosmetic use:

- More than any other product, foundation makes the most difference in boosting one's overall attractiveness, according to studies that have surveyed men. This is because it smooths the skin and makes users appear "healthier."
- Women have another take on the matter. In scientific studies involving women, they found females wearing eyeliner, eye shadow, and mascara to be the most beautiful. They also considered women who wear makeup to be more dominant and strong.
- Red is the most universally attractive shade of lipstick and is preferred over brown, nude, and other shades. Pink is runner-up. Why red? It creates contrast, which is pleasing to the eye.
- Painting one's nails can be therapeutic and has been scientifically proven to boost both calmness and overall mood.

Makeup use can also make one feel smarter. A study titled "The Lipstick Effect" showed that more than positive music or looking at positive images, wearing makeup caused participants to see themselves as more capable. With this boost of confidence came much higher test scores.

However, scientific studies have also shown that there is such a thing as "too much makeup." A research study published by Kramer & Ward had participants take three photos. In the first photo, they were wearing no makeup. In the second, they were wearing a moderate amount of makeup. For the third photo, they were instructed to apply their makeup as if they were going out for the night. For the first stage of the study, a panel of non-participants (both male and female) judged the photos. The results were unanimous: both sexes preferred the moderate look and thought the women were less attractive with a full-face of cosmetics. Interestingly, the participating women in the photos actually thought they looked better with the "full-face."

## COSMETICS AND CHEMISTRY

Today, cosmetics can be defined as products created to protect, cleanse, or change the way our outer bodies look or feel. One of the most scientific things about cosmetics is the way that they are created—through **chemistry**! When you think about chemistry, the periodic table and lab experiments are probably what come to mind, but at its most basic level, it is the study of substances. This is what cosmetic science is all about.

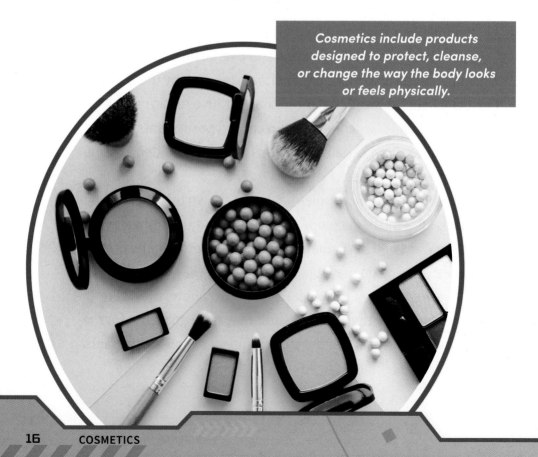

*Cosmetics include products designed to protect, cleanse, or change the way the body looks or feels physically.*

# A BOOMING BUSINESS

The beauty industry is a global one. Worldwide, 100 billion dollars a year is spent on makeup, perfume, skincare, and hair products. Americans spend more money on cosmetics than they do on education and use an average of 11 products per person every day. The industry continues to expand, experiencing a 7 percent increase in growth between the years 2014 and 2015, putting it at a similar level to huge industries such as apparel and jewelry.

So far, we have only discussed makeup and skincare, but it is important to note that cosmetic products include those created for application to the teeth, underarms, and other parts of the skin. These are sensitive areas, so it is important that chemists ensure that the cosmetics are created keeping in mind both use and safety. After all, we wouldn't want a Venetian ceruse repeat.

There are hundreds of thousands of cosmetic products marketed for sale, so it is not practical to list the thousands of ingredients used. In the United States alone, there are more than 12,000! Although the formula for each product created changes slightly, most cosmetic products contain some mixture of the following eight core components: water, preservatives, thickeners, **emollients**, emulsifiers, fragrance, color, and pH stabilizers.

The process of creation is different for each chemical formula. A vast majority has emollients (lipids) as a base. Common emollients include shea butter, mineral oil, paraffin, beeswax, lanolin, or coconut/olive oil.

# EMULSION

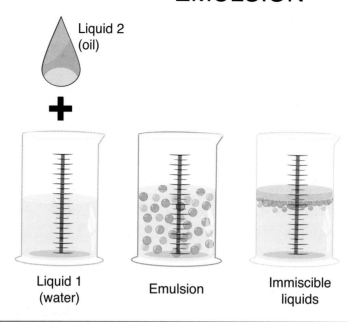

Liquid 2 (oil)

**+**

Liquid 1 (water)

Emulsion

Immiscible liquids

*Emulsions are a combination of two substances that do not mix naturally.*

**Emulsions** are also common in cosmetics. Emulsions are made up of ingredients that are chemically incompatible, such as oil and water. Emulsifiers help keep these incompatible components from separating. Homogenized milk is a typical example of an emulsion, where the fat does not separate as it naturally would. Borax with beeswax is an often-used emulsifier. Adding a pH stabilizer helps keep emulsions stable and on the shelf for a longer period of time.

In many cosmetic labs, thickeners are added to some products, usually in the form of wax or polymer. Cosmetic chemists also use preservatives to keep what they have created from being overrun by bacteria, yeast, and mold. Many microbes live in water (a key ingredient in most cosmetics), so there has to be something to keep the products from being taken over by microorganisms. The most common are parabens and para-aminobenzoic acids, but others are used as well.

*Biophysicist Luca Turin explains the molecular makeup that gives a perfume its scent.*

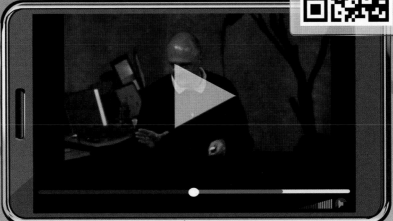

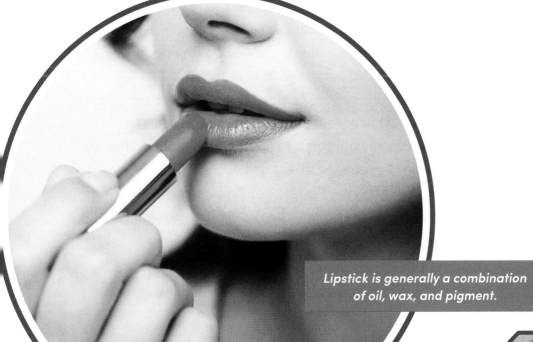

Lipstick is generally a combination of oil, wax, and pigment.

# PUCKER UP! LIPSTICK FACTS

The very first lipstick was created more than 4,000 years ago in the Middle East. In those days, women ground up precious stones and gems and used the dust for lip decoration. Today, lipstick is made in a different way. Although there are many variations, all lipsticks are a combination of oil, wax, and pigment. Differences in dryness (alcohol), preservatives, fragrance, and color make each tube slightly different from others on the market.

In recent years there has been a big push for cosmetic companies to be more accountable when it comes to ensuring that the ingredients they are using in their products are safe. Although there are more than 1,000 common cosmetic components that are considered toxic, only 11 are illegal in the United States. For this reason, it is important to avoid chemicals of concern. For help with what to look for, a quick Google search for a cosmetic chemical "red list" will help you weed out the good from the bad.

The connections between cosmetics and science are amazing. Just as the use of beauty and body care products helps to shape our culture, mindset, and approach to physical appearance, they are also influencing how we see others and ourselves. By learning more about the link, we can have a better understanding of how using various products can impact our lives and the world around us in a positive way.

# TEXT-DEPENDENT QUESTIONS

1.  What do people in the field of cosmetic science study?
2.  Name one psychology-based, scientific finding related to cosmetics.
3.  What are the four key components found in most cosmetics?

# RESEARCH PROJECT

A cosmetic company has hired you as a researcher and product developer. Your task is to create a product that solves a common beauty problem. What would you create and why? List the ingredients and some simple steps you'd use to make your invention. Also, list a few that you would make sure to leave out.

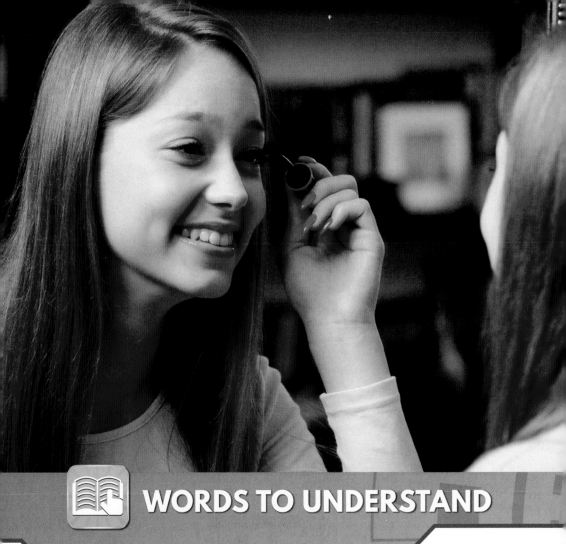

## WORDS TO UNDERSTAND

**algorithm**—a group of rules or a procedure created to solve a particular problem, especially by a computer

**artificial intelligence (AI)**—the capability of a machine to simulate intelligent human behavior

**astigmatism**—an eye condition in which irregularly shaped corneas make vision blurry

**augmented reality (AR)**—a reality-based, computer-generated environment that uses technology to enhance a user's real-world experience

# CHAPTER 2

# TECHNOLOGY
## IN COSMETICS

Technology has made a notable impact on the cosmetic industry as we know it today. Technological advancements in **artificial intelligence (AI)**, **augmented reality (AR)**, and other areas have made it possible for manufacturers of cosmetics to personalize products in new ways. As a result, cosmetic users are now able to make strides toward achieving their desired outer appearance using a customized and unique approach. In a world that is moving closer and closer to individualized routines in beauty, the demand for product offerings like these is likely to grow with each passing year.

## SKINCARE TECHNOLOGY

Skincare is a prevalent and lucrative part of the cosmetic industry. Globally, the skincare market raked in almost $135 billion dollars in 2018. Over the course of the last 10 years, that represents an increase of nearly 60 percent. A big part of the reason why the skincare industry has seen this type of growth is due to the technological advancements made available over the course of

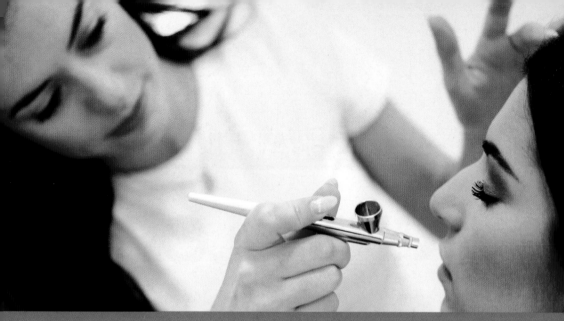

*Makeup artists often use an airbrush to apply foundation because the technique provides even coverage and a natural, finished look.*

the last decade. Without this growth in technology, it is possible virtually no growth might have occurred and the industry may have become stagnant. When cosmetic industry leaders take initiatives to continually discover the next "big thing," it encourages engagement and excitement within the industry, which in turn boosts growth even more.

Airbrushed models on the covers of major magazine publications and in televised advertisements have set a standard for radiant, glowing skin. The role of skincare technology in cosmetics is to help consumers achieve the best-looking skin possible for them. Some of these technologies are designed to analyze individual skin types and formulate regimens or specific products to achieve a person's desired look. In today's society, people are moving further and further away from a "one-size-fits-all" approach to skincare. In response, skincare giants like L'Oreal have developed specific applications and software to cater more toward providing a personalized experience for each and every user.

# Smart Serums

The demand for personalized skincare products has led one manufacturer to create special smart serums. These serums from Clinique (a division of the self-named American cosmetics company created by Estée Lauder in 1946) are made up of thousands of different combinations and are specifically formulated for the user that requests them. Small stickers armed with sensors are attached to the user's skin and collect information on sebum level, oiliness, pH level, and much more. Then, this data is used to create a unique serum to fix any skin problems that are detected.

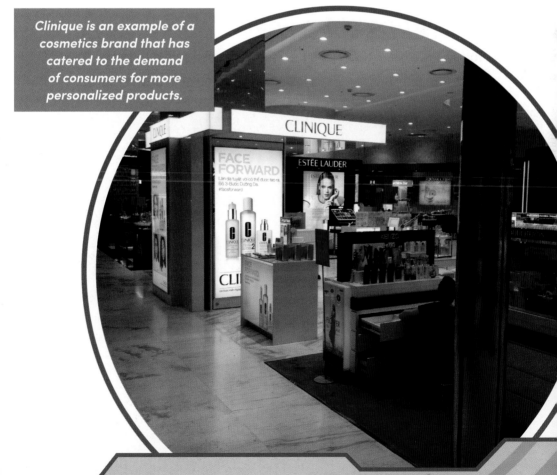

*Clinique is an example of a cosmetics brand that has catered to the demand of consumers for more personalized products.*

An **algorithm** is then used to detect any skincare changes over time. This means that the more consumers use the product, the more in tune the serum will be with their skin. In other words, as the skin changes, the formula does too. The technology for algorithms like this has been around for decades and is used to identify user preferences on social media platforms like Facebook and entertainment video streaming services like Netflix. This just goes to show that the demand for services specifically catered to each individual is being met across many different platforms and therefore enforces the idea that cosmetic providers need to move in the same direction to stay in touch with consumer expectations.

## Skincare and Genetics

Today, we already have the technology to use saliva to get information about ancestry using DNA. If you search the online

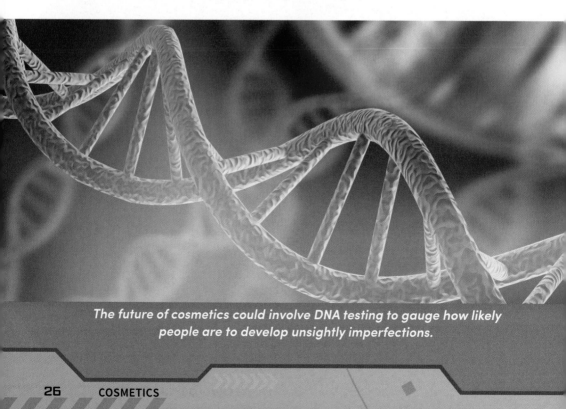

*The future of cosmetics could involve DNA testing to gauge how likely people are to develop unsightly imperfections.*

marketplace, you can easily find saliva collection kits that can collect genetic material that can then be tested to determine ancestral lineage. This same technology has the potential for innovating the cosmetic industry in a big way. Since these tests already have the capability to detect certain genes that make us more susceptible to certain diseases and other ailments, they could be manipulated to calculate the possibility of deep wrinkles, varicose veins, and various other perceived cosmetic imperfections as we grow older.

In the future of cosmetics, this data could be used to get valuable insight into how we might expect to age over time. It can then be used to design skincare regimens that diminish the effects of aging by predicting the probability that proteins like collagen will be underactive or overactive as users begin to grow older. Then, formulas can be produced to fight (and maybe even prevent) the effects that cause reactions that make us appear older. For example, vitamin C has been shown to have positive effects on collagen when used over time. If a person's saliva swab shows that they are at risk of collagen breakdown, cosmetic products with vitamin C as an active ingredient could be prescribed to help combat this condition. Although we haven't quite reached the point where this can be executed yet, it is probable that it is coming in the next decade or so.

## Automated Skincare Machines

A beauty brand in Japan called Shiseido launched an innovative skincare machine in 2019 called Optune. Users begin by scanning their faces into an app and answering some basic questions about their skincare routine and skincare goals. Then, the app consolidates this information and the company uses it to customize special cartridges loaded with cosmetic products. These cartridges are then loaded into a special machine that dispenses the perfect amount of product for each application. The machine also detects when users are low on product and automatically orders more cartridges when necessary.

This skincare machine meets several demands of cosmetic consumers today. The first is the demand for specialized beauty products that are tailored to the user. The second is a "set-it-and-forget-it" approach to ordering products. The online retail marketplace in the United States had revenues of about $2.8 trillion dollars in 2018, and those numbers are expected to grow to a whopping $4.8 trillion dollars by 2021. With such a large amount of revenue running through e-commerce sales, it makes sense that cosmetic companies would focus product distribution in this arena.

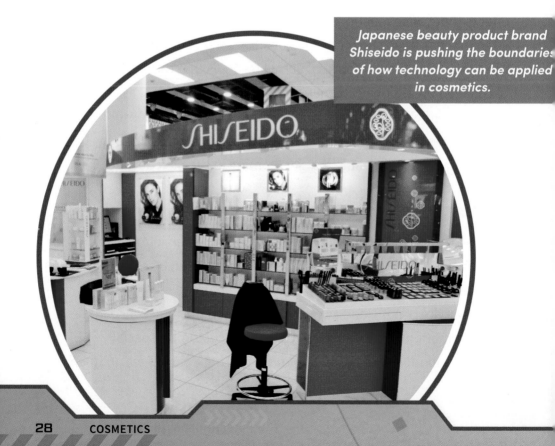

*Japanese beauty product brand Shiseido is pushing the boundaries of how technology can be applied in cosmetics.*

The best part about this approach is that some people can eliminate the need to see a skincare specialist to address their needs. As long as no severe reactions are present, the application paired with the specialized approach to skincare will be enough to solve problems for most consumers without ever stepping out of their front door. The convenience factor is sure to save a lot of time and effort on the part of cosmetic consumers around the world.

## Artificial Intelligence and Skincare

AI is a great example of how technology has transformed the way skincare is approached today. AI has been integrated into software programs and applications and has even been used to

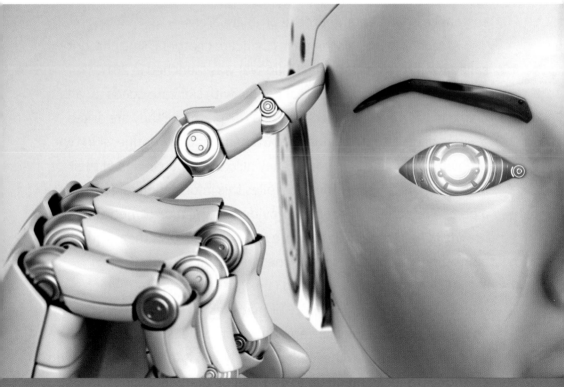

*Like it is in several industries, AI is increasingly used in relation to cosmetics.*

# ARTIFICIAL INTELLIGENCE

Hollywood movies often depict AI by telling stories about robots that develop real human emotions and either save or plot to destroy the world. The reality of AI is that it is simply a computer program that is given a specific job to do. Engineers and other product developers sometimes work many years to compile all the information needed to build a good AI machine.

create beauty treatments. These AI-designed products work by analyzing abnormalities on the skin's surface, such as dark spots and hyperpigmentation. Then, they use this information to formulate a custom cosmetic to target these problem areas.

AI technology is also used for skincare chatbots. One chatbot called Ava (from tech startup HelloAva) was launched in 2017. It works by interacting with real people with skincare needs on an online platform. When users log in to the platform, they are asked a series of targeted questions about their skincare routine, skin type, problem areas, and skin goals. They also submit an image of their face. The AI technology then compiles this information and provides a personalized list of products provided by trusted cosmetics brands to help zero in on skincare issues and resolve them with the appropriate products that give the best results possible.

CEO Grace Choi co-founded Mink (as in Makeup Ink), which released a makeup printer in 2019 that uses AI to color match any image uploaded to the Mink app on your mobile device. The app connects wirelessly to the Mink printer, which is loaded with makeup cartridges that can blend up to 16.7 million different shades. In just 15 seconds, the printer prints the image in makeup onto specially designed makeup sheets. The product is then applied directly from the sheet. This creates the ability to exactly match the tone of a user's face. This technology would simplify and automate the process of choosing makeup. Consequently, users could have makeup that perfectly complements their skin each time they use the product and could save the cost and time needed to hire a professional who could provide similar results. This is just another example of how technology in the cosmetic industry is empowering consumers to take charge of their own routines.

The first working AI programs were developed in the 1950s to play checkers and chess. Now, smart home devices such as the Amazon Alexa that use this technology are in millions of homes. The technology is still being developed and perfected along the way, which suggests that even bigger things may be possible in the future.

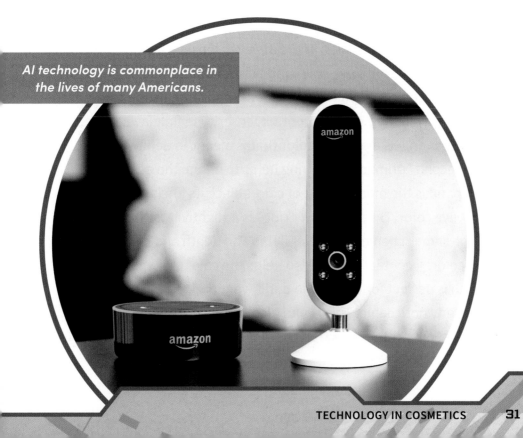

*AI technology is commonplace in the lives of many Americans.*

Although AI's application to makeup might not be as flashy as futuristic robots, it has the potential to revolutionize the industry as we know it.

# TECHNOLOGY AND CONTACT LENSES

Technology has transformed the way we think about contact lenses today. In previous years, these lenses have been utilized as an alternative to eyeglasses but didn't have any non-aesthetic benefits. As technology has progressed, contact lenses have evolved. Nowadays, contact lenses can be worn for cosmetic effects even if you don't need a prescription to help you see.

While contact lenses do serve as a medically necessary product, they can also be considered a cosmetic item. Especially since most of the time, glasses can be worn for the same vision-enhancing effects that contacts offer. There are even lenses that have the ability to change a person's eye color and pupil shape as well.

FreshLook, a popular contact lens innovator, uses a three-part technology in their colored contact lenses. The first layer, called the outer ring, is a primary color that is meant to define the eye. The second "primary color" ring helps to define the desired eye color and is the most vibrant of colors since its job is to transform your eye color. The final "inner ring" is a slightly less vibrant color in the same scheme. This layer helps add depth and definition to the colored contact lens. It also helps the color look more natural, which is perfect for those who don't want their contact lenses to be overly noticeable. This brand also carries more subtle versions of the same contact lens that has similar layers, but each of them is

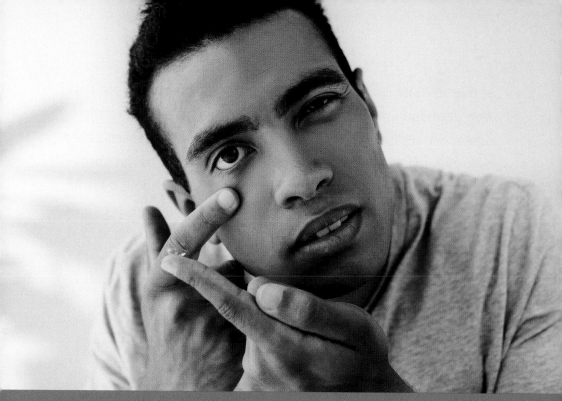

*Although vision correction is the prime use of contact lenses, in many cases they can also be viewed as cosmetic.*

less saturated for a subtler look, which is great for people who prefer to enhance their natural eye color rather than to transform it completely.

Recent technologies in the contact lens industry have also made it easier than ever for people with certain eye conditions to get a pair of contacts that will work for them. SynergEyes, for instance, is a hybrid contact lens whose technology makes it possible for people with severe **astigmatism**, irregular corneas, and certain eye diseases to get contacts. People with conditions such as these might not have an option to get contact lenses if it weren't for technological advancements that have made it possible today.

In the past, people who needed bifocals to read and also have astigmatism only had two options: to wear special glasses in addition to their contact lenses or to opt for more rigid, gas permeable lenses. New developments in contact lens technology have changed the scenario for these people—there are now soft contact lenses, called toric multifocal lenses, which allow people who have astigmatism and presbyopia to see from a distance and to read without difficulty. This is a big plus for people who don't like to wear glasses because they don't have to sacrifice their appearance in order to see as best they can.

# AUGMENTED REALITY TECHNOLOGY

**Augmented reality** applications and advertisements are the latest and greatest in the cosmetic industry. According to a report completed by Zion Market Research, the AI industry that we have today will be worth close to $133 billion by 2021. This is largely due to the changing preferences and behaviors of consumers in the modern day. In other words, technologically advanced beauty products are on a steady rise and that trend is expected to continue as time goes on.

Since new polls have shown that millenials spend more time interacting on their phones than in the real world, it makes sense that an AR approach would appear in the beauty industry. There are AR applications that can be used to virtually "try on" makeup, access beauty tutorials, get vital product information, and more. As more technological advances are made, capabilities are likely to grow above and beyond these uses. This means that the makeup industry, as we know it today, may be vastly different as soon as a few years from now.

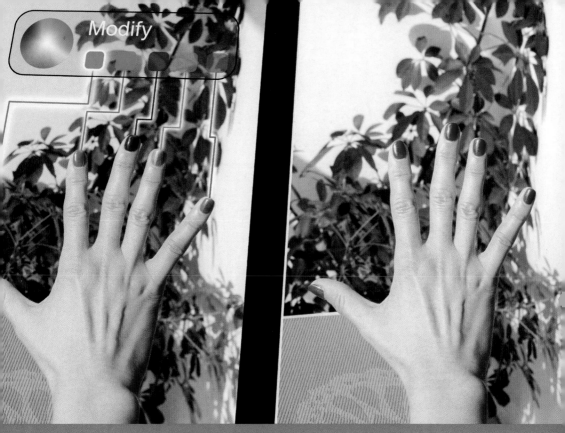

Modify

With augmented reality technology, trying on different shades of nail polish takes just seconds.

Augmented reality is changing the way that online shoppers think about the cosmetic industry. In the past, people who shopped online for cosmetic products such as makeup and nail polish had no way of knowing how a certain item would look on them. Since there is often a wide variety of shades and formulas to choose from, it would be difficult for people to make an informed decision on which products to purchase from online retailers. AR technology makes it possible for anyone to have a good idea of what to expect from a product before it comes in the mail. The cosmetics portion of online revenue accounts for more than a billion dollars worldwide, and this option opens doors for even more growth in the future and a better experience for those who shop online.

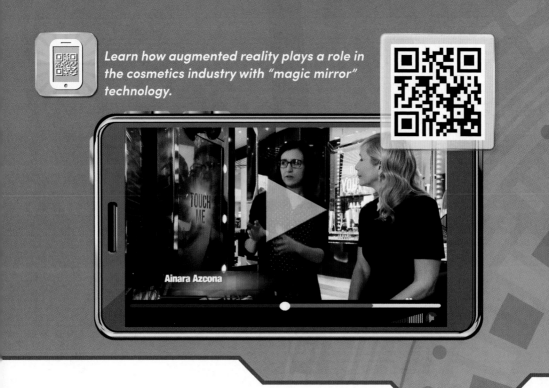

Learn how augmented reality plays a role in the cosmetics industry with "magic mirror" technology.

Ainara Azcona

# BEAUTY PRODUCT TECHNOLOGY

As the demand for technology in our daily lives rises, so does the demand for high-tech beauty products. In response, several beauty brands have released products that help people reshape their beauty regimens by using technology.

Many of these products combine the technologies discussed in previous sections for the ultimate user experience. One example is smart mirrors. These mirrors first utilize AI to analyze a user's skin. The data collected in this step can help give users advice about what makeup products to use and tips on how to best apply them. This allows users a more interactive and user-friendly experience to makeup, especially for those new to the cosmetics game.

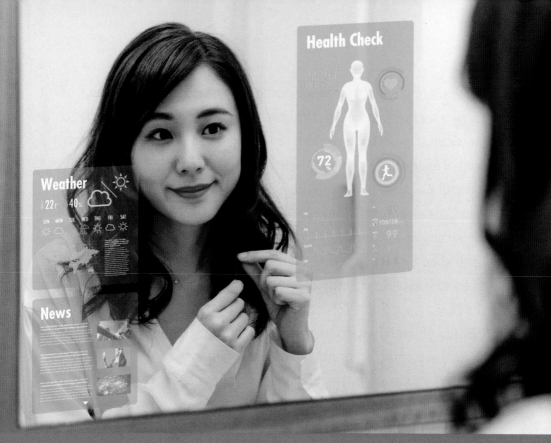

*Smart mirrors give information, but they can also take it by running an analysis of the user's skin.*

Then, users have augmented reality to allow them to try on the day's makeup virtually before they even begin their routine. Just like creating a character in a video game, users can literally try on different looks with the swipe of a finger. This simplifies the process of getting ready in the morning, saving precious time for users, allowing more time to spend on the things that really matter like eating breakfast with the family or getting to school in time to catch up with friends before the first bell.

These high-tech mirrors could also be helpful in brick and mortar retail chains that sell makeup. Imagine you are shopping for makeup and you see a brand of cosmetics that runs thirty shades of lipstick. You have narrowed your favorites down to your top 10, but you are having trouble deciding which one to buy. The lack of current technology inside the store means that we would have to physically try on each option, removing one color before trying the next. Depending on the pigment within each lipstick, this could be difficult because of residue from the previous shade, and harshly rubbing the area to remove multiple shades could also be irritating, physically and mentally. AR mirrors could allow you to see how each shade looks on you in a matter of seconds. It eliminates the need to waste time applying and removing shades, and it makes the buying process simpler and more straightforward for everyone. Instead of spending hours inside the store picking the perfect shade, you could be done in a matter of minutes and walk out with the perfect shade for the occasion of your choice.

High-tech cosmetic products aren't only present in the skincare and makeup world. L'Oreal recently released a smart hairbrush that boasts some pretty cool technology too. This special brush was designed to analyze the user's hair and give detailed feedback about it. This information is used to recommend specific products to improve the health of hair and to enhance healthy hair brushing routines and processes. These smart hairbrushes achieve this by sending alerts when users brush hair too quickly or roughly. They also have tiny microphones and other sensors that detect hair breakage and otherwise weak areas. The technology within these brushes allows users access to data about their hair health and care routines in a way that has not been possible before. Since hair is considered a hallmark of beauty for many people, women and men alike, it is a real asset to have access to this information to enhance and specialize a hair care routine.

Each of these smart beauty devices serves a specific purpose in every user's life, and the capabilities available are expected to get more and more complex. The detailed information that most of these apps and machines provide helps users become more knowledgeable about how to care for themselves and put their best foot forward.

## 3D PRINTING IN COSMETICS

3D printing has been around since the early 1980s, but it has gained traction in the cosmetics world much more recently in the

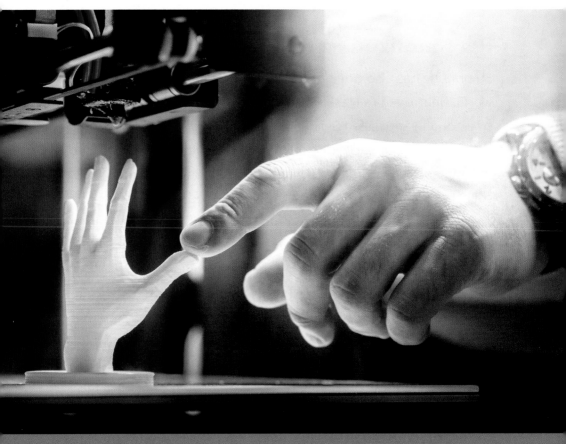

*To improve its efficiency, the cosmetic industry is getting a helping hand from 3D printing technology.*

early 2000s. 3D printing has now made it possible to manufacture beauty products such as mascara wands and enabled packaging to be done quicker and more efficiently. Although this method of production and innovation has a long way to go before it is perfected, it is still helping the cosmetic industry to make strides toward a brighter future. It will do this by simplifying and expediting the production process, making the packaging less expensive, and thereby lowering costs to consumers and even helping to customize consumers' cosmetics experience with personalized face masks, customized makeup palettes, and more.

## Personalized Face Masks

3D printing has also transformed personalization in the beauty world. Neutrogena's MaskiD combines this technology with their smartphone app called Skin 360. Originally, this app allowed users to scan their faces into a program that would make product recommendations with its technology based on information collected. Now that 3D printing has been added into the mix, customized face masks that contour exactly with a person's face are made available to the public as well.

We are all individuals, and no skincare product has universal success across all people. Face masks that are tailored to specific users fortify the cosmetic industry because users can be sure that the product that they use will work for them. This eliminates the need to buy and try multiple products before finding the right fit. The notion that this process can be completely skipped is likely a part of the reason why consumers today are so drawn to custom cosmetic products and tools.

# 3D Printing and Cosmetic Packaging

3D printing has the potential to create endless shades of makeup in the future (we will talk more about this later), but in the present day, it has made a considerable impact on the packaging side of cosmetics. The 3D printer makes it easy to design and make prototypes of cosmetic packaging, which cuts down on time used to create these designs. It also nearly eliminates the chance of design flaws and errors during the manufacturing process. This means a ton of saved money for cosmetic suppliers and potentially lower-cost products for consumers.

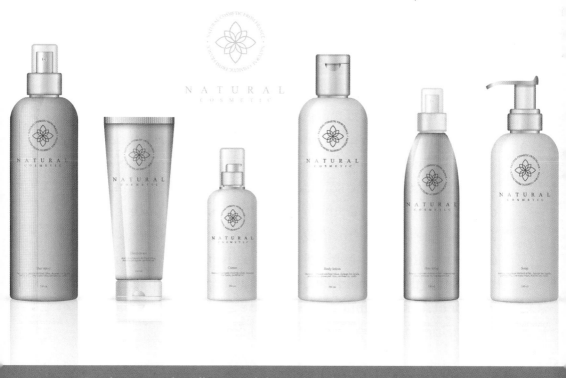

*3D printers can handle even elaborate packaging, which drastically cuts the production costs.*

Perhaps the most notable industry segment that 3D packaging printing impacts is luxury makeup, which typically has more elaborate packaging. This is because of the preciseness of the printing process. Manufacturers can now 3D print perfectly sharp and detailed packaging without the hassle of going through the drawn-out prototyping process.

At the end of the day, an automated and simplified production process means a more successful cosmetic industry. The time spent designing and prototyping new packaging could be better spent on developing new formulas or technologies to catapult the industry into further success. Less waste equals more money to innovate and engineer new products as well.

## The Future of 3D Printing in Cosmetics

Although the technology isn't quite perfect yet, there is some potential for 3D-printed makeup to be available in the future. Since anything thicker than milk cannot go through a 3D printer on its own, solvents would need to be used. Then, users would have to wait a few hours for the solvents to evaporate before the makeup could be used. However, this method still has value, since it would allow people to create their own custom shades of makeup and unique palettes to fit their individual needs. There is also some speculation that it would eliminate single-use plastic packaging in favor of reusable options that would mesh better with this personalized approach to creating makeup.

# TEXT-DEPENDENT QUESTIONS

1. What is artificial intelligence?
2. What are some examples of high-tech beauty products?
3. Who co-founded Mink?

# RESEARCH PROJECT

Technology has become a part of the cosmetic industry in a big way. Locate and try out at least three different applications that have been designed to enhance a consumer's experience with cosmetics. These can be smartphone applications, websites, or any other technology-based platform built with cosmetics in mind. Then, create a list of pros and cons for each application or website.

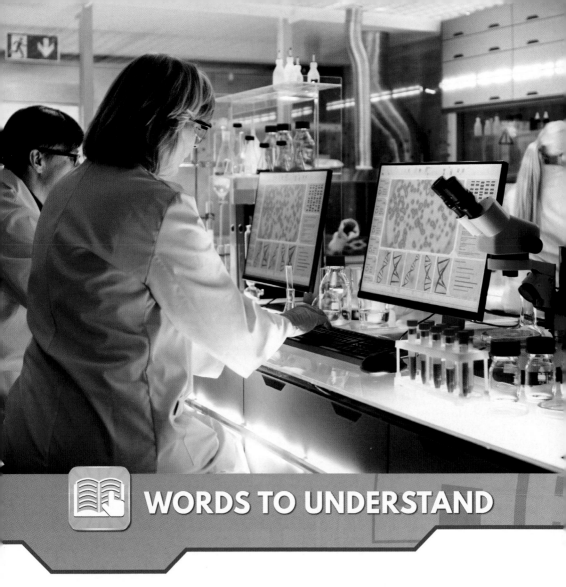

**benchmark**—something that serves as a standard by which others may be measured or judged

**formula**—a combination of ingredients that make up the components of a cosmetic item

**organic**—naturally occurring products or ingredients that come from living matter

**vetted**—having been subjected to evaluation or appraisal; critically reviewed and evaluated for official approval or acceptance

# CHAPTER 3

# ENGINEERING
## IN COSMETICS

A chemical engineer is an essential part of any cosmetics operation. Most of the time, the people who hold these roles are college-educated professionals who take their jobs very seriously. It is important that they do so because their role is to protect the public from mistakes in manufacturing that might cause illness, skin rash, or other side effects. These engineers are also responsible for ensuring the best possible product results from the manufacturing processes they oversee. Without a chemical engineer spearheading the processes at any lab, the cosmetics on the market today would be questionable at best. You can thank the engineering process for the level of quality in the products you have come to know and love.

## ENGINEERING AND COSMETICS

Many people might think that chemical engineering is mainly a sector of the oil and gas industry. While chemical engineering is an important part of oil and gas, it is useful in cosmetics, as well. If you have ever read the back of a bottle of shampoo, you probably know that the percentages of different elements are listed there.

The engineering process ensures that these ingredients are stored properly when they arrive at production facilities, they are broken down properly when it is time to combine them, and they are handled properly when being added into the formulations for the cosmetics that we are familiar with and have come to love.

As the demand for **organic** cosmetics within the beauty market grows, so does the need for chemical engineers. This is because the combination of organic ingredients requires staff members with a strong background in understanding the naturally occurring ingredients that organic cosmetics include. Many man-made ingredients are designed to have a long shelf life, which prolongs the amount of time they can be stored before they are used. Fabricated ingredients are also created to be especially hardy when handled. This helps to avoid waste if they are handled improperly.

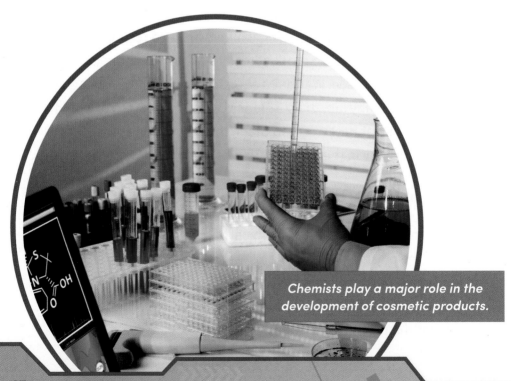

*Chemists play a major role in the development of cosmetic products.*

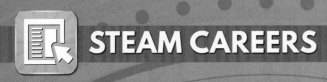
Cosmetic items such as makeup and skincare products aren't a simple science project. The ingredients that make up these items are carefully combined and then rigorously **vetted** before they even make it to a testing phase. The process of combining and testing each element along the way requires years of experience. A person that gains this experience and applies it to cosmetic production is called a cosmetic chemist. Cosmetic engineers create and oversee the entire process that cosmetic chemists will need to execute in order to make the highest quality product possible.

Chemical engineers also play an important role in deciding how to handle raw products that will be used in their **formulas**. Most of the time, cosmetics companies order these ingredients in bulk because they need to produce large amounts of product at a time. A chemical engineer can analyze these materials and give crucial insight into how they should be handled or stored for the best results. This helps ensure the ingredients in our makeup and other cosmetic items remain safe and healthy for regular use. It also helps ensure that products maintain a stable shelf life, and it can even determine certain temperatures that products can endure without being damaged or destroyed.

Without having a chemical engineer as part of any production line, there might not be anyone to hold accountable for the handling of raw materials in the assembly line. However, the most important skill that an engineer in this industry must possess is the ability to work with a team effectively. The functions of an engineer are only made possible if there are chemists and lab technicians to perform the jobs assigned to them by the engineers. In general, the role of a chemical engineer is

# A RECIPE FOR SUCCESS

When it comes to organic components, the handling process must be refined. Since these elements are derived from natural sources, they have little to no protection against poor handling or storage techniques. A chemical engineer can determine the specific needs of each organic property and can create a process that will best preserve the components of each one. Think of this process as a recipe—if the ingredients aren't handled properly, and the instructions aren't followed in the correct order, you will end up with a dish that could make someone sick or won't look as appetizing as it should have.

important, but in the cosmetics and beauty world, he or she plays an even bigger role.

Most chemical engineers in the cosmetic industry work in special cosmetic laboratories and are responsible for creating the products that we see on the shelves in stores. Since cosmetics are chemically formulated products that help people look their best, chemical engineers are vital in the production process of all cosmetic products.

Whether it is colognes, perfumes, makeup, skincare products, or anything of the like, chemical engineers create the formula. Their job is to test certain combinations of ingredients to see if the result is a safe, effective, and useful product. They also work very closely with other members of cosmetic production teams such as market researchers and planners, to align their formulations with the goals and vision of the company they work for.

*Check out this look at a day in the life of a cosmetic chemical engineer.*

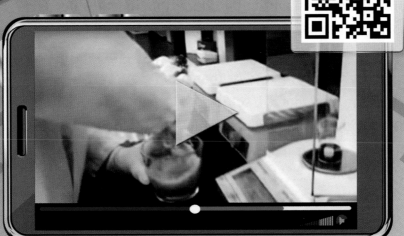

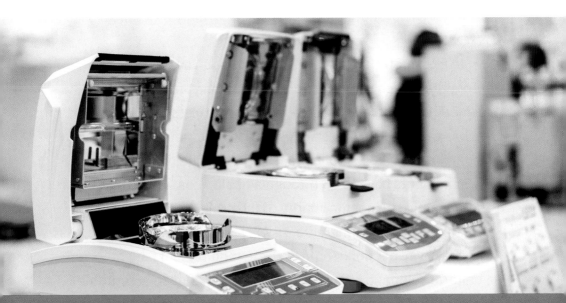

*Each ingredient that goes into a cosmetic formula is precisely measured, some with high accuracy scales such as those shown here.*

Chemical engineers are a vital part of the supply chain for a number of reasons. First, they have the know-how needed to produce well-thought-out products that meet the needs of consumers from all different backgrounds. They also provide much needed structure in the production environment. This structure ensures high-quality products that stand the test of time and are worth the money they are sold for. This helps give the cosmetic industry a glowing reputation that in turn, helps it succeed and continue to grow as it has for many years before and many years still yet to come.

## The Role of Engineering in the Production Process

We know that the job of a cosmetic chemist is to mix and test certain ingredients that make up the cosmetics we use in our every day lives. The production process is full of many other processes as well.

In a cosmetic lab, ingredients go through several stages before they reach their final form. Depending on what type of cosmetic product is being created, these processes will vary, but the basics of each process are essentially the same. Once all of the ingredients are compiled for the product being produced, the ingredients have to go through a quality control process. The cosmetic engineer in charge of the project determines what **benchmarks** the raw ingredients will have to meet in order to pass this quality inspection. Some of these requirements might include a uniform color and shape, a pleasant smell, and an acceptable temperature. Cosmetic chemists inspect these products to ensure they are within the set standards, and once approved, they send them on to the next stage in development.

Once the ingredients for any product pass the vetting process, they will move into either the production stage or the storage stage. During this part of the process, it is imperative that chemists, lab technicians, and any other person who comes into contact with raw ingredients is properly trained on how to handle them correctly. It is the job of a chemical engineer to decide what these rules should be. Engineers will use their education and prior job knowledge to determine these rules and will enforce them, often with the support of industry executives.

A chemical engineer can help find out and explain how to handle the goods in either process. For the production stage, special gloves or other equipment might be needed in order to maintain the

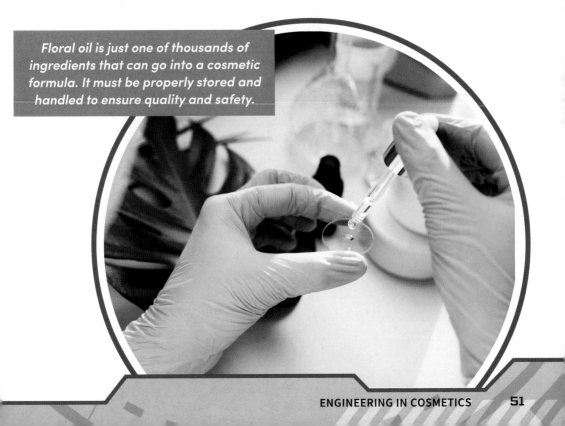

*Floral oil is just one of thousands of ingredients that can go into a cosmetic formula. It must be properly stored and handled to ensure quality and safety.*

quality and potency of certain ingredients. During the storage stage, certain temperatures, storage techniques, and shelf-life information might be considered most important. The overseeing chemical engineer is usually the first person to determine the standards set for each of these stages and is also charged with making any changes necessary along the way if a certain step in the process fails.

If the chemical engineer creates a process that works well, the end result should be a product that is as close to perfection as possible. For most engineers, this means setting strict rules and processes surrounding the entire production period. Rules also help simplify the production process since they provide a road map to follow for any processes to be completed during the production chain. Without a cosmetic engineer, all of this may not be possible.

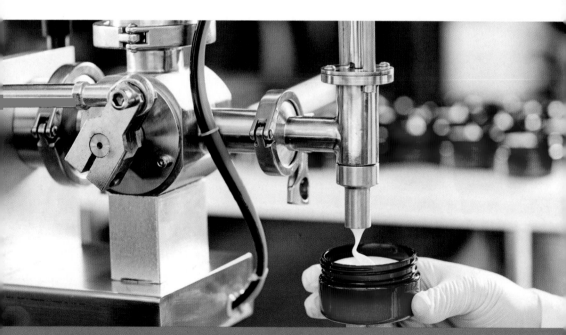

*If all procedures are strictly followed, the end cosmetic product should be close to perfect.*

**TEXT-DEPENDENT QUESTIONS**

1. What is the main role of a cosmetic chemical engineer?
2. Why is it important that cosmetic ingredients are handled properly and combined according to the regulations of chemical engineers?
3. True or False: A role of a cosmetic chemical engineer is to ensure cosmetic products are produced in a way that they will be safe, effective, and useful to the consumers who purchase them.

 **RESEARCH PROJECT**

Imagine you are a chemical engineer at a major beauty company. Your boss has just told you that you are being assigned to create a process for making a new lipstick. What steps should be taken from start to finish to create this product? What are some best practices you would tell chemists to have? What are some things chemists would have to stay away from? Combine all your data onto a poster board and show it to the class. Extra points for creativity!

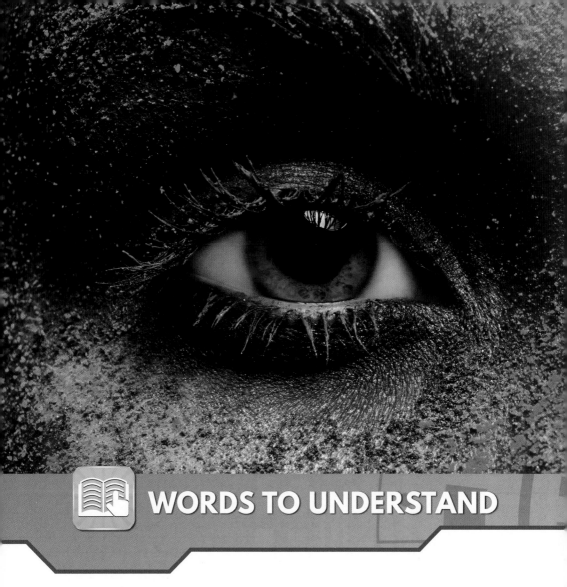

## WORDS TO UNDERSTAND

**henna**—a reddish-brown colored paint made from a tropical plant native to certain areas in Africa and Asia

**color theory**—a set of principles that determines how to mix colors for the best-looking outcome

**connoisseurs**—people who understand the details, technique, or principles of an art and are qualified to act as critical judges; experts

# CHAPTER 4

# ART
## IN COSMETICS

At the heart of body painting and makeup application, you will find artistry. Even though these applications may not look like art on the surface, there is often artistic intention behind each stroke of the eyelash brush. People use body paint and makeup to express themselves, to make a statement, and to look their best visually. This chapter will go over the history of certain cosmetic art, how it's relevant, and how it has the power to change lives.

## BODY ART

Evidence of body art traces all the way back to the origin of mankind. Body painting in particular was used by people in ancient times to show their status, their religious beliefs, and even to protect themselves against evil or disease. In these times, brightly colored paints foraged from berries and other naturally occurring substances were used on the face and body.

In today's world, body paint is still used by some tribes and cultures to indicate changes in life, such as getting married. A tradition in India called Mehndi is a notable example of body art in modern times. This process involves using **henna** paints to create intricate designs on a woman's hands and body to celebrate her wedding. These henna paints can last up to 12 weeks and are an example of a natural body paint that is used in modern society. This is a tradition that traces back thousands of years and has continued on due to cultural expectations in the country.

Body paint has also been used to communicate artistic vision in recent times. One example of this occurred in the hippie era of the 1960s. Since this movement embraced sexuality and nudity, many people took the opportunity to express their artistic visions by decorating the female body. Then in August 1992, the cover of Vanity Fair magazine featured a photo of actress Demi Moore wearing nothing but body paint. Body paint in these two instances was used to create a buzz in the media and to shock people who witnessed them, but it is important to note that the unclothed female body is not the only place where body paint is displayed in modern times. It can also be present on smaller parts of the body and with clothing.

Body paint can also be used to make a statement. Political and social protesters associated with PETA, an animal activist group, have used body paint as a way to gain public attention in support of their cause.

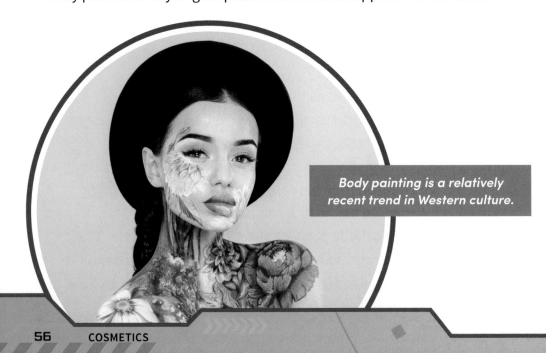

*Body painting is a relatively recent trend in Western culture.*

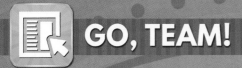

# GO, TEAM!

If you have ever watched a professional football game, you have probably seen mega fans in the audience with brightly painted faces and bodies reflecting their team's colors. This is a form of body art! These fans are so passionate about their team that they literally painted their team's colors on their bodies for all to see. Talk about team spirit!

Activists have created full-body looks impersonating tigers, dead fish, and even the skeletons of people to make their voices seen and heard. These shocking images are intended to garner public attention and therefore bring attention to group initiatives.

Instead of using a canvas, some artists choose to create their art solely on the human body. One artist in China, Liu Bolin, uses body paint

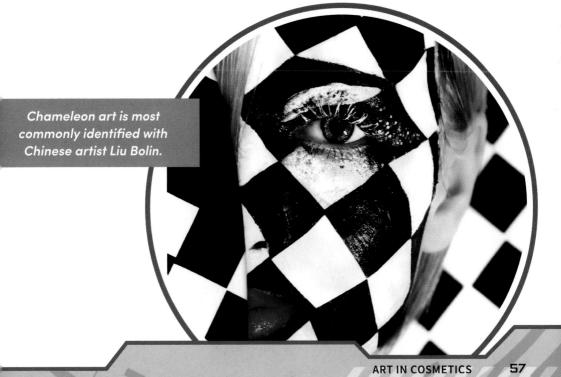

*Chameleon art is most commonly identified with Chinese artist Liu Bolin.*

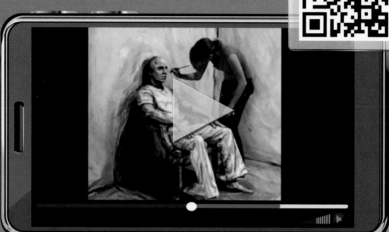

*Artist Alexa Meade shares her experience using the human body as a canvas in her TED talk.*

on himself to create works of art. He is commonly known by the name "Invisible Man" because he uses body paint to camouflage himself into his surroundings like a chameleon. As with most art, Bolin's work has a vision behind it. After the city that he was working in was destroyed, he was moved to create his first series of chameleon art. This was done with the intention of drawing attention to artists who receive little to no support from the Chinese government—almost as if they are invisible.

Body art can also be used to create optical illusions. Alexa Meade is an artist who uses her artistic abilities to paint the human body to appear one-dimensional. Meade uses people as her canvas of choice because it helps her creativity flow with more fluidity and passion. She is not inspired by one-dimensional canvases and has said that there is much to be desired when working with them. The complexity of the human body inspires her to create images that challenge the mind with enticing optical illusion.

# COLOR CORRECTION

Color correction is a cornerstone of makeup and cosmetic artistry. In an environment where makeup is used, color correction is needed to cancel out discolored areas on the body such as red spots, dark areas, and scars. Makeup artists often use green, coral, or purple concealers underneath flesh-colored foundations to cancel out any unsightly skin blemishes. The result is a more even-toned skin appearance and therefore a more beautiful canvas to work with when applying makeup to other areas of the face.

In the hair care industry, color correction is also very important. We have all seen the movie depictions of a bad dye job—the scene where the main character goes into a salon looking to go bleach

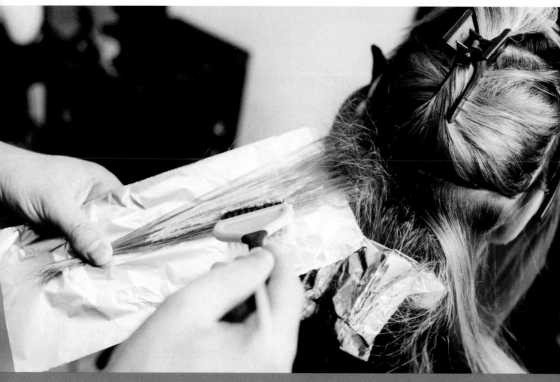

*Color correction accounts for a huge amount of business in the hair care industry.*

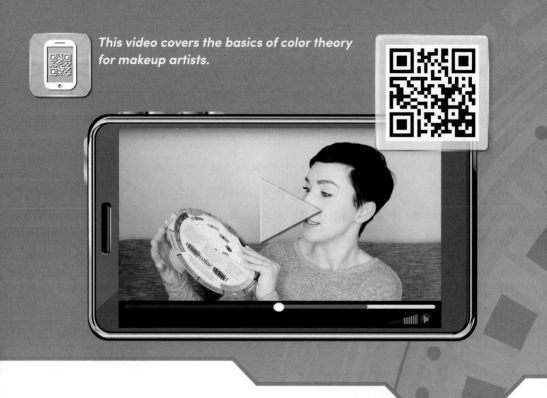

*This video covers the basics of color theory for makeup artists.*

blonde but instead ends up with bright green locks. This situation represents real-life scenarios where color correction is needed. Professional hair stylists assess the hair color and use **color theory** to determine what should be done to correct the damage done. We will talk more about color theory later in this section.

## BEAUTY TOOLS

Much like any typical artist, makeup artistry uses a wide variety of key tools to achieve their artistic vision. Makeup brushes, sponges, and many other tools of the trade are necessary to execute any successful makeup look. Although these makeup enthusiasts aren't working with oil pastels and acrylic paints, they are still artists in their own rite. Their intention is to create a beautiful work of art that is pleasing to the eye, has its own mood, and might even be a statement for all to see.

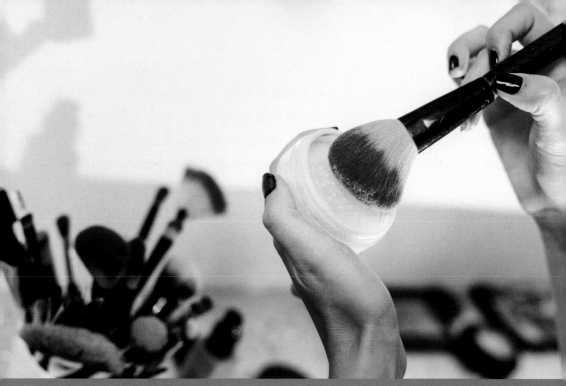

*Knowing when to use which brush is part of the skill set of makeup artists.*

Makeup artists use brushes of all different shapes and sizes to do several different jobs. Some of these include applying eye shadow, highlighting cheekbones, and setting the foundation with a fine powder. These makeup brushes also range in material. Many of these brushes are made with synthetic fibers, but there are varieties that include natural animal hair as well. Makeup artists decide which type of brush to use based on the application. If a product application needs to look dense and saturated, a synthetic brush is the best option. For more natural-looking applications and gradients, animal hair does the best job. Most makeup applications require a combination of both types of brushes and specific knowledge about which products work best with which brushes— both are essential to any successful makeup artist's arsenal. Just like an artist with a brush, makeup artists must know their medium and know it well if they hope to succeed.

Beauty sponges are employed in a few different ways as well. The most current trend for using beauty sponges is for applying foundation. While a special foundation brush can also be used for these applications, a beauty sponge boasts a more natural-looking and smooth finish versus a brush. These sponges can also be used to apply powder to certain areas when highlighting and contouring the face. Makeup artists strategically use this tool to blot the powder underneath the eye to set concealer and at the base of the jawline to make the contour pop and look much sharper and neat.

Various other tools, such as eyelash curlers and eyebrow spoolies, are also used to achieve the artistic vision of makeup artists and clients. These tools work on perfecting small hairs and making eyelashes look taller and more defined. Although perfection isn't always necessary when it comes to applying makeup, having a well put together appearance normally is. When makeup artists take the time to ensure no hair is out of place, it exemplifies this in a big way. Just like artists, makeup **connoisseurs** in this rite ensure that their work is as presentable as possible before showing it off to the world.

## MAKEUP ARTISTRY

The art of makeup is the subject of many social media posts and YouTube videos. There are tutorials on practical makeup looks, transformations for Halloween, date nights, holiday parties, and much more. On the opposite end of the spectrum, many makeup enthusiasts and makeup artists create futuristic-looking landscapes and abstract works of art on their faces. There are even people that use lipstick to paint murals on their lips! This just goes to show that there are endless amounts of self-expression within the makeup industry that proves the artistry of it all.

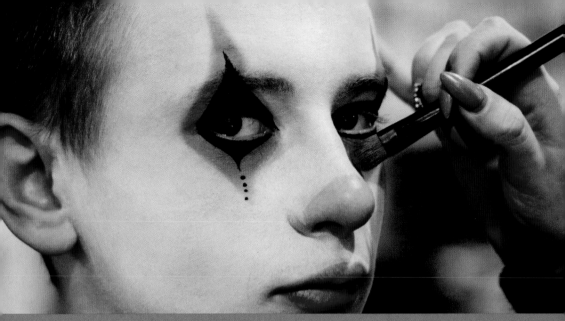

*Makeup artists are skilled at creating looks from the practical to the terrifying or comical.*

In cosmetics stores today, eye shadow palettes and lipsticks come in just about every shade that you can think of. This enhances a user's ability to create colorful, artistic works of art on their faces and bodies. Within makeup artistry, there are several artistic elements to keep in mind.

## Line Work

Line work is one facet of makeup that contributes to the artistry of the end result. For example, creating "winged" eyeliner is a trend that is widespread across the beauty world today. This look is achieved by using special cosmetic products called liquid eyeliners. Liquid eyeliners are applied wet using precise brushes or felt-tipped pens.

Line work knowledge is also important to have when applying other products to the face and other areas of the body. A popular trend called contouring and highlighting involves adding slightly darker shades to certain parts of the face such as the hollows of the cheeks and the outer edges of the face and lighter or shimmery shades to "high points" like the tops of the cheekbones and the tip of the nose. This is done with the goal of making a face look more ovular – a highly coveted face shape sported by models and celebrities. Understanding where the lines on the face are located is essential to knowing where to place products strategically.

## Shading

Just like in traditional art, shading plays a vital role in makeup application. This principle is mainly used when applying eye shadow. Most modern makeup looks call for a gradient look when applying the shadow to the eyes. Makeup artists must understand how to properly shade each color in order to get the desired effect.

Shading is also important to artistic applications like Halloween and abstract looks. This is especially true when bright colors are involved because if they are not shaded correctly, colors might blend together unintentionally, which could result in a muddy or unorganized look.

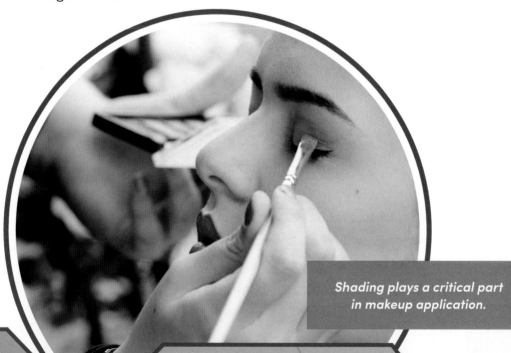

*Shading plays a critical part in makeup application.*

## Color Theory

Color theory plays a role in makeup artistry across the entire canvas of the face. When deciding on colors to use in any makeup application, colors that complement one another must be used for the most aesthetically pleasing result. Much of the time, makeup artists will match warm colors with like colors. Some with a more artistic vision may mix colors, but they must still pay attention to color if they want to maintain a sharp look across the face or body.

## Theatrics

If you have ever seen a movie, you've witnessed first-hand the result of a makeup artist's job. Filmmakers require a dedicated team of artists to create the environment needed to film a movie. For films that are set in the past, rigorous research must be done to determine what trends in makeup and other cosmetic features are needed to be

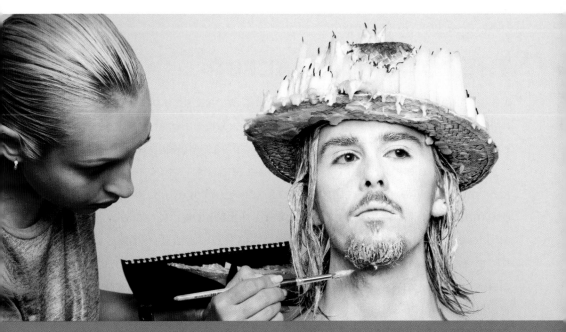

*From movie sets to the Broadway stage, makeup artists are a critical part of creating the world directors are imagining and by which audiences are enthralled.*

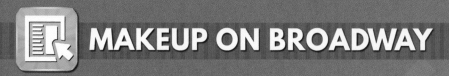

Theatrical production teams have makeup artists on staff. The makeup used for theater workers has to be able to withstand the heat from spotlights and other equipment used on stage, so special makeup that is resistant to these conditions is used.

true to the era. This is also true for movies about a person's life. When an actor is depicting a real-life person, makeup artists must depict them in a way that is true to the real person they are playing. The role is so crucial that the Academy of Motion Picture Arts and Sciences in Hollywood gives a coveted Academy Award (known as an Oscar) to the best makeup artist in the industry each year. The most successful Hollywood makeup artist is Rick Baker, who won seven Oscars for movies such as *Men in Black* and *How the Grinch Stole Christmas*.

## THE POWER OF MAKEUP

Makeup has the ability to have a dramatic impact on a person's life. When makeup artists use their artistry to enhance the natural features of their clients, they are truly transforming their canvas. Makeup looks range from simple to extravagant. Both women and men can use makeup to look more awake, more refined, and better put together. Women often use makeup to make their eyes appear brighter, their faces look sharper, and to diminish imperfections such as skin flaws and dark bags under the eyes. Men also commonly use makeup for the same purposes but can also gain a sharper-looking jawline or brow bone. Children can even take advantage of the artistry by becoming fictional characters on Halloween or sporting red lipstick and sparkly eyelids for cheer events or dance recitals. When it comes to makeup, the possibilities are endless.

# TEXT-DEPENDENT QUESTIONS

1. What is henna?
2. Which beauty tool is often used to achieve a smooth and natural look when applying foundation?
3. Why is color theory important to makeup artists?

# RESEARCH PROJECT

Do an online search for an artistic makeup look or body paint model. What do you think the artist was trying to communicate to the audience when he or she created it? If you were the artist who created the look, what would you have included, or what would you have removed? Share your findings with the class.

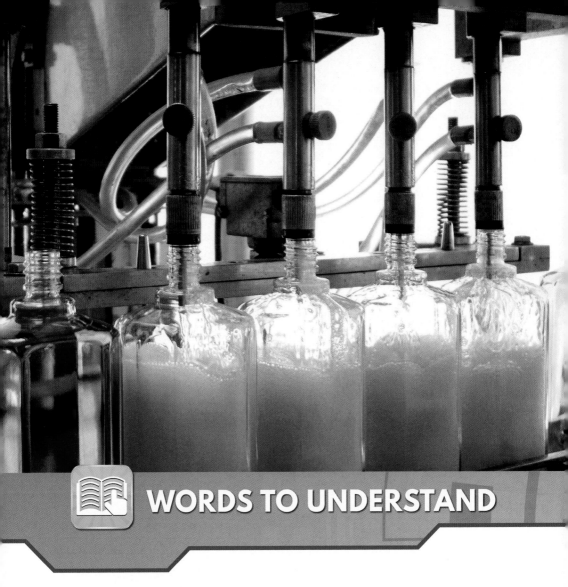

## WORDS TO UNDERSTAND

**active ingredient**—in regard to cosmetics, the portion of a solution that is made up of the raw form of any ingredient

**geometry**—a branch of mathematics that deals with shapes

**symmetrical**—two parts of one whole that are exactly the same on each side

# CHAPTER 5

# MATH
## IN COSMETICS

Cosmetics and math are two things that go hand in hand. This relates to the cosmetic manufacturing process where products must be measured and to the makeup artistry sector where people use makeup to make their faces look more **symmetrical**. This chapter will go over beauty standards and how they relate to math in the cosmetic industry.

## MATH AND COSMETIC CHEMISTRY

Whether we are talking about makeup, skincare products, perfumes, or hair dyes, they all have one thing in common: a formula. Math in cosmetics starts with the chemistry of these formulations and how each ingredient adds up to make the final product. There are several steps in this process.

The first step to formulate any cosmetic item is calculating the percent of activity in each ingredient. When ingredients arrive in manufacturing plants, they are often delivered as a raw

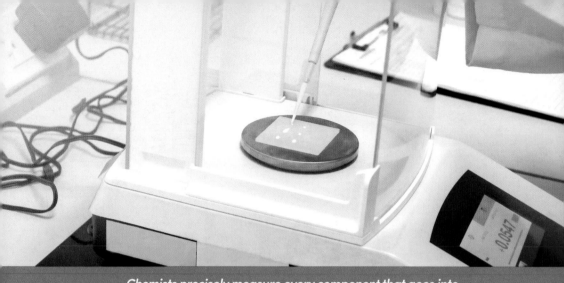

*Chemists precisely measure every component that goes into a cosmetic product's formula.*

material dissolved in water. A cosmetic chemist must then use a mathematical formula to figure out what percentage of the solution contains the **active ingredient** and what percentage is water or other elements. Next, it is time to create the chemical formula for any given product. This involves combining the raw ingredients together and ensuring that the proper proportions are used.

The initial batch created by the formula that chemists start with is usually not large enough to support mass production. If this is the case, the next step is to scale the formula by multiplying the number of ingredients in the smaller batch to make the recipe for a larger batch. This is done using another specialized formula that helps determine the number of raw materials that must go into a recipe to yield enough product overall.

The last step chemists take in producing cosmetics is converting units. In the lab, all the numbers in each math equation are figured using the metric system. When the formula reaches its final stages, it is necessary to convert these measurements into the imperial units still used in the United States. Multiplying the mass or volume of grams or milliliters by the relevant conversion factor completes the process.

*Cosmetic chemist James Neil demonstrates how he makes beauty brand ColourPop popular lux lipsticks.*

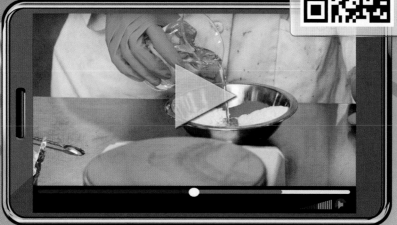

# SYMMETRY: THE MATH THAT DETERMINES BEAUTY

One of the main goals of cosmetic products is to make people look and feel more beautiful, or at least more aesthetically pleasing. This might not seem to have much to do with math, but it does.

Scientists have proven that people are more inclined to recognize other people as more beautiful the more symmetrical their features are. In fact, there is a mathematical "golden ratio" that many believe is the key to determine whether a person is beautiful or not. This ratio is based on the Fibonacci numbers, named after the 12th century Italian mathematician. The Fibonacci numbers make up a sequence in which every third number is the sum of the previous two (i.e., 0, 1, 1, 2, 3, 5, 8 and so on). If you continue down the line and express the numbers as a ratio by dividing each by the one preceding it

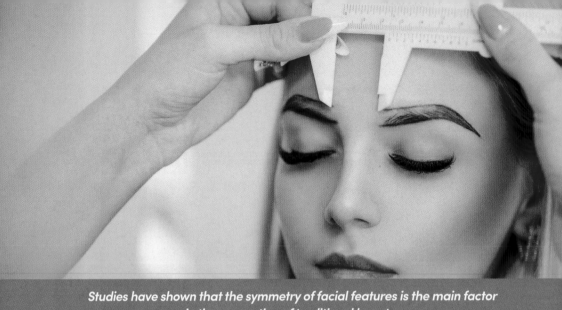

*Studies have shown that the symmetry of facial features is the main factor in the perception of traditional beauty.*

(i.e. 8/5), you end up with a number that mathematicians call "phi," an irrational number that goes on infinitely (1.61803 …). The ratio 1:phi is the golden ratio and phi is the universal number for beauty because it appears recurrently in nature and has been used to construct many "beautiful" structures such as Michelangelo's "David" statue.

But how does this all relate to cosmetics? The idea behind the math of cosmetics is that makeup can be used to make a face and body look more symmetrical. As mentioned in the previous section, contouring and highlighting the face and body can help make both sides look alike to one another. Therefore, the closer the symmetry of each side of the face or body, the more beautiful a person will appear.

Dr. Kendra Schmid, chair of the College of Public Health, Department of Biostatistics at the University of Nebraska Medical Center, developed a scale based on 29 measurements of the face that generates a beauty score, where 10 is perfect. The first measurement is the length of the face divided by the width of the face. For the most attractive people, that answer is phi, or 1.6 times longer than it is wide. The other measurements are of additional

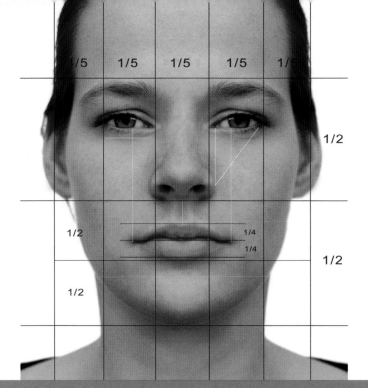

1/5 1/5 1/5 1/5 1/5

1/2

1/2 1/4

1/4

1/2

1/2

*The prevailing theory is that the closer each side of the face measures to the other, the more beautiful it is perceived to be. Used effectively, makeup can help to balance any asymmetry.*

features such as the distance between the eyes should equal the width of one eye, the nose should be the same length as an ear, the mouth should be twice as wide as it is full, etc.

Cosmetic surgery can also help people with asymmetrical faces to look more beautiful. Injections like Botox and Juvaderm help people plump areas of their faces on each side until a near-perfect match is achieved. These injections are not permanent; so they require ongoing upkeep, but for those who want to maintain as symmetrical a face as possible, it is an option.

## MATH IN HAIR CARE

Math also plays an important role in a hair care environment. If you have ever had your hair professionally colored in a salon, you know that cosmetologists use unique dyes to help you achieve

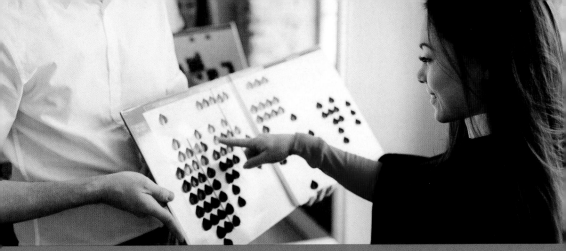

*Hairstylists and cosmetologists all use math to take care of their customers' hair.*

your desired look. Did you know that the dye used on your hair is combined using math? Your hairstylist uses math to decide how much dye to use to saturate your hair and which colors to mix together to achieve your desired hair color.

Math in hair care doesn't stop there. **Geometry** and math are used to determine what haircuts would work best for you and what formulations of product to use to keep your hair looking the best. Even the deep conditioning treatments that you have applied at the salon must be measured accurately if you hope to get the best results.

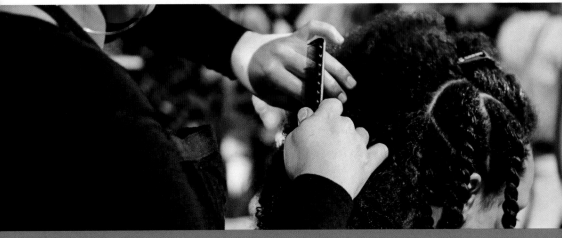

*Hairstylists use geometry to make sure your style looks just right.*

# TEXT-DEPENDENT QUESTIONS

1. What is an active ingredient?
2. What is the golden ratio?
3. Which cosmetic injections are commonly used in surgery to make a face appear more symmetrical?

# RESEARCH PROJECT

Consider the role symmetry plays in how beautiful a person might appear to others. Then, draw a picture of a symmetrical face and asymmetrical face side by side. Record your thoughts on each. Which one do you find more appealing? What could be done to the asymmetrical face to make it appear more aesthetically pleasing?

# FURTHER READING

Amparo, Salvador. *Analysis of Cosmetic Products 2nd Addition*. Amsterdam: Elsevier Science, 2017.

Hernandez, Gabriela. *Classic Beauty: The History of Makeup.* Atglen: Schiffer Publishing, 2017.

Rayma, Marie. Make it Up: *The Essential Guide to Makeup & Skin Care.* Philadelphia: Running Press, 2016.

Sakamoto, Kazutami, Robert Lochhead, Howard Maibach, and Yuji Yamashita. *Cosmetic Science and Technology: Theoretical Principles and Applications*. Amsterdam: Elsevier Science, 2017.

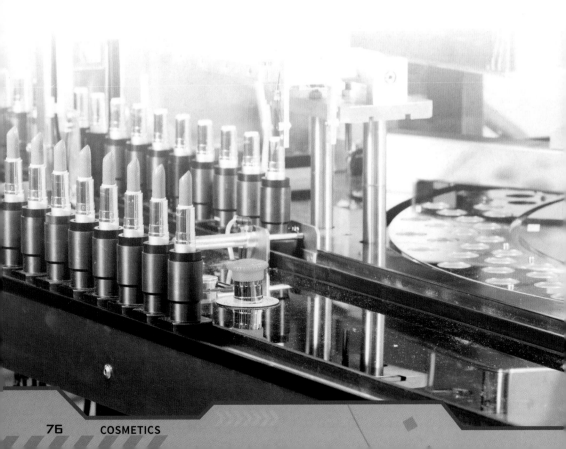

# INTERNET RESOURCES

*https://cosmeticsinfo.org*
A website that explores the relationship between science and cosmetics in modern-day applications.

*https://www.aiche.org/conferences/conference-on-engineering-cosmetics-and-consumer-products/2019*
This website includes publications about the role engineering plays in the cosmetic space.

*https://www.laurahendersonmakeup.com/beauty-blog*
This resource contains valuable information about the art of makeup and how makeup artists apply certain products to enhance the beauty of their clients.

*https://www.scconline.org*
The Society of Cosmetic Chemists' website includes journals and resources dedicated to the advancement of cosmetic science

*https://chemistscorner.com/math-used-in-cosmetic-product-formulation*
A resource explaining the role that math plays in a cosmetic production operation.

# EDUCATIONAL VIDEO LINKS

*Chapter 1: http://x-qr.net/1KMR*

*Chapter 2: http://x-qr.net/1KNx*

*Chapter 3: http://x-qr.net/1Ku3*

*Chapter 4: http://x-qr.net/1Jhy*

*Chapter 4: http://x-qr.net/1J0d*

*Chapter 5: http://x-qr.net/1LVe*

# INDEX

# AUTHOR BIOGRAPHY

Mary Elizabeth Dean is a teacher and author who is passionate about writing books that not only educate but also inspire. Her ultimate desire is to encourage all types of kids to find their own unique path and life's purpose. As a Louisiana transplant by way of Tennessee, Mary enjoys trips to New Orleans, reading forgotten classics, and hunting for treasures in thrift stores with her children.

# PHOTO CREDITS